Nourish: A Comprehensive Guide to Optimal Health Through Nutrition

BY ANDREW R. McLean

Copyright © 2023 by Andrew R. McLean

All rights reserved

 No part of this book may be reproduced, distributed, or transmitted in any form or by any means, including photocopying, recording, or other electronic or mechanical methods, without the prior written permission of the publisher, except in the case of brief quotations embodied in critical reviews and certain other noncommercial uses permitted by copyright law.

For permissions requests, write to the publisher at
AndrewRMcLean@dayrep.com

Table of Contents

- **Embracing Lifelong Healthy Eating Habits**

Chapter 1: Introduction

Welcome to the captivating journey of "Nourish: A Comprehensive Guide to Optimal Health Through Nutrition." In this inaugural chapter, we set the stage for an exploration that will not only deepen your understanding of nutrition but also revolutionize the way you approach food and well-being.

Section 1: The Vital Role of Nutrition in Health

Imagine a world where every bite you take is a step toward a healthier, more vibrant you. In this section, we delve into the profound impact that nutrition has on every facet of our lives. Beyond mere sustenance, the food we consume is the fuel that powers our bodies, drives our energy levels, and lays the foundation for our overall well-being.

Embark on a journey through the intricate web of cellular interactions and metabolic processes, where nutrients are the currency of life. Uncover the remarkable influence of nutrition on the body's ability to heal, regenerate, and thrive. From strengthening our immune systems to supporting organ function, the vitality of every cell hinges on the nutrients we provide through our dietary choices.

Section 2: Understanding the Basics of Nutrients

Prepare to be amazed by the symphony of nutrients that orchestrate our bodily functions. In this section, we embark on a voyage into the microscopic world of vitamins, minerals, carbohydrates, proteins, and fats. These fundamental building blocks are more than just words on a label; they are the keys to unlocking our potential for optimal health.

Dive into the intricate dance of macronutrients and micronutrients, each playing a vital role in the grand symphony of life. Uncover the magic of carbohydrates, those energy-packed molecules that power our every move. Explore the awe-inspiring world of proteins, the architects of our muscles and tissues. And venture into the realm of fats, those misunderstood heroes that cushion our organs and fuel our brains.

But this chapter is just the beginning. As we journey deeper into "Nourish," you'll not only learn about the components that make up our food but also gain the tools to wield this knowledge for your well-being.

So fasten your seatbelt, for the voyage into the heart of nutrition has only just begun.

Chapter 2: The Foundation of a Healthy Diet

Welcome to a culinary odyssey through the heart of nourishment! In this chapter, we will embark on a captivating exploration of the foundational principles that underpin a vibrant and balanced diet, transforming the way you think about the food on your plate.

Section 1: The Five Major Food Groups: A Palette of Nutritional Diversity

Imagine your plate as a canvas, waiting to be adorned with a rainbow of nutrients. In this section, we delve into the symphony of flavors and colors that make up the five major food groups. Each group represents a unique reservoir of vitamins, minerals, and essential nutrients that contribute to your overall well-being.

As we traverse the vibrant landscapes of fruits and vegetables, we discover that their colors hold the key to their nutritional prowess. From the regal purples of berries to the earthy greens of leafy greens, each hue signifies a treasure trove of antioxidants and health-promoting compounds.

Step into the realm of grains, where the humblest of seeds transform into nourishing staples like bread, rice, and pasta. Learn the art of selecting whole grains that offer sustained energy and a wealth of fiber, supporting digestive health and satiety.

Venture further to the protein realm, where animal and plant-based sources await to fortify your body's structure. From the lean grace of poultry to the versatility of legumes, discover a multitude of options to cater to your nutritional needs.

And let's not forget the dairy and dairy alternatives, those sources of calcium and vitamin D that empower your bones to stand tall. From creamy yogurts to nut-based milk, explore choices that align with your dietary preferences.

Section 2: Portion Control and Balanced Eating: The Symphony of Satisfaction

Prepare to unlock the art of portion control, where the balance between sustenance and satisfaction is masterfully maintained. In this section, we delve into the intricacies of serving sizes and the role they play in achieving and maintaining a healthy weight.

Explore the mindful practice of savoring each bite, as you cultivate a deeper connection with the food on your plate. Discover how portion distortion can distort our perception of serving sizes and lead to overeating, and learn strategies to recalibrate your sense of portion adequacy.

Embark on a journey to create balanced meals that honor the wisdom of moderation. Dive into the world of macronutrient ratios, discovering the magic of combining carbohydrates, proteins, and fats to create a harmonious culinary experience.

And as we navigate this chapter, remember that balance is not just a nutritional concept; it's a mindset. It's about honoring your body's needs while also indulging in the pleasures of food. So take your time, relish each moment, and let the symphony of flavors and nutrients nourish not just your body, but also your soul.

Chapter 3: Exploring Macronutrients: Unveiling the Building Blocks of Vitality

Prepare to embark on an epic expedition into the heart of macronutrients, those powerful building blocks that shape your energy, strength, and overall well-being. In this chapter, we will unravel the intricate tapestry of carbohydrates, proteins, and fats, discovering their profound impact on every aspect of your life.

Section 1: Carbohydrates: The Fuel that Ignites Your Fire

Imagine carbohydrates as the energetic spark that propels you through life's adventures. In this section, we delve into the dynamic world of carbohydrates, from the simplest sugars to the complex structures that provide sustained energy.

Journey through the spectrum of carbohydrates, from the rapid surge of glucose to the gradual release of complex carbs that keep you fueled for hours. Explore the magical interplay between simple and complex carbs, learning how to harness their powers to enhance athletic performance and maintain steady blood sugar levels.

Delve into the intriguing realm of dietary fiber, those indigestible marvels that promote digestive health and provide a lasting sense of fullness. Learn the art of selecting high-fiber foods that support weight management and reduce the risk of chronic diseases.

Discover the art of carbohydrate timing, uncovering how pre- and post-workout meals can optimize your exercise performance and recovery. With carbohydrates as your energetic allies, you'll be ready to conquer any challenge that comes your way.

Section 2: Proteins: The Architects of Your Inner Universe

Prepare to meet the architects of your body, the proteins that construct and repair tissues, hormones, and enzymes. In this section, we explore the dynamic world of proteins and their indispensable role in every facet of your physiological existence.

Dive into the fascinating world of amino acids, the intricate puzzle pieces that form the protein mosaic. Learn the difference between essential and non-essential amino acids, and how your dietary choices influence their availability.

Discover the balance between complete and incomplete protein sources, understanding how different foods contribute to a symphony of amino acids that sustain your muscles and promote growth. Delve into the fascinating world of protein quality, as we explore the concept of biological value and the power of plant-based proteins.

Venture into the world of protein synthesis, where the body's master builders translate dietary protein into functional structures. Explore the science behind muscle repair and growth, and uncover strategies for optimizing your protein intake to support your fitness goals.

Section 3: Fats: The Unsung Heroes of Vitality

Prepare to be captivated by the enigmatic world of fats, those essential molecules that not only fuel your body but also play a crucial role in protecting your organs and maintaining cellular function. In this section, we embark on a voyage into the realm of fats and their intricate roles in your health.

Uncover the truth about dietary fats, dispelling myths and embracing the diverse array of fats that nature offers. Learn to distinguish between saturated, unsaturated, and trans fats, understanding how their chemical structures influence their impact on heart health and overall well-being.

Journey through the omega-3 and omega-6 fatty acids, those powerful agents that regulate inflammation, support brain function, and contribute to cardiovascular health. Explore the sources of these essential fatty acids and learn how to achieve a balanced intake for optimal health.

As you navigate this chapter, remember that macronutrients are more than just numbers on a nutrition label; they are the tools that shape your physicality, influence your energy levels, and support your journey toward vibrant health. So savor every bite, honor the diversity of nutrients, and let the magic of macronutrients become an integral part of your nourishment narrative.

Chapter 4: Micronutrients and Their Impact: Unveiling the Hidden Heroes of Health

Get ready to plunge into the microscopic realm of micronutrients, those silent superheroes that wield an incredible influence over your health and well-being. In this chapter, we embark on an illuminating journey through vitamins and minerals, uncovering their secrets and unraveling their roles in every aspect of your body's functions.

Section 1: Vitamins: The Alphabet of Wellness

Imagine vitamins as the alphabet of wellness, with each letter representing a unique role in maintaining your body's harmony. In this section, we delve into the world of vitamins, exploring their diverse functions and understanding how their absence or abundance can shape your health.

Embark on a tour of vitamin-rich foods, discovering how fruits, vegetables, and other dietary sources are brimming with these essential nutrients. From the immunity-boosting power of vitamin C to the vision-enhancing qualities of vitamin A, learn how each vitamin contributes to your body's intricate symphony.

Explore the antioxidant prowess of vitamins like E and C, as they shield your cells from the ravages of free radicals and promote cellular health. Delve into the roles of B vitamins, those energy-boosting agents that keep your metabolism humming and your nervous system firing on all cylinders.

Section 2: Minerals: The Silent Architects of Life

Prepare to uncover the silent architects of life, the minerals that regulate bodily processes and maintain structural integrity. In this section, we journey into the world of minerals, discovering their roles in maintaining electrolyte balance, promoting bone health, and supporting countless physiological functions.

Dive into the essentiality of minerals like calcium and magnesium, those powerhouses that empower your bones and muscles to stand tall and strong. Explore the dynamic interplay of sodium, potassium, and chloride, which regulate fluid balance and nerve transmission.

Delve into the intricate world of trace minerals, those enigmatic elements like zinc, selenium, and iodine that play small roles but wield significant influence. Learn about their functions in immune support, antioxidant defense, and thyroid health.

Section 3: Nutrient Synergy: Where Vitamins and Minerals Dance

Prepare to witness the intricate dance of nutrient synergy, where vitamins and minerals collaborate to amplify their impact. In this section, we explore how these micronutrients work together in harmonious ways, enhancing absorption, utilization, and overall effectiveness.

Delve into the art of pairing foods that naturally complement each other, creating meals that optimize nutrient absorption. Discover how vitamin C can enhance the absorption of non-heme iron from plant-based sources, and how vitamin D supports calcium utilization for bone health.

Explore the fascinating world of food synergy, where whole foods offer a symphony of nutrients that work in tandem to nourish your body. Learn how a colorful salad isn't just a feast for the eyes but also a celebration of nutrient diversity and harmony.

As you navigate this chapter, remember that micronutrients are the unsung heroes that fuel your cellular machinery, regulate your biochemical processes, and support your long-term well-being. So explore the diversity of vitamins and minerals, honor their synergy, and let the intricate dance of micronutrients become an integral part of your health narrative.

Chapter 5: Building Healthy Habits: Cultivating a Lifetime of Nourishment and Wellness

Welcome to a transformative chapter that invites you to lay the foundation for lifelong well-being. In "Building Healthy Habits," we delve into the art of planning and preparing meals, crafting smart snacking strategies, and cultivating a holistic approach to nourishment that will guide you on a path of sustainable health.

Section 1: The Blueprint of Success: Mastering Meal Planning and Preparation

Imagine meal planning as the blueprint of your nutritional success, guiding you toward balanced and nourishing choices. In this section, we embark on a journey into the world of meal planning, discovering how this powerful practice can streamline your dietary journey.

Explore the benefits of planning ahead, from saving time and money to reducing stress and ensuring balanced nutrition. Dive into the art of creating weekly meal plans that reflect your dietary goals and preferences, all while keeping your energy levels steady throughout the day.

Venture into the world of batch cooking and meal prepping, unlocking the secret to effortlessly assembling wholesome meals on even the busiest days. Learn to wield portion control as a tool for mindful eating, creating meals that satisfy your hunger without overindulgence.

Section 2: Smart Snacking: Navigating Between Meals with Purpose

Prepare to redefine the way you snack, transforming those in-between moments into opportunities for nourishment and energy. In this section, we explore the art of smart snacking, where every bite serves as fuel to sustain you throughout the day.

Delve into the science of satiety, understanding how protein and fiber-rich snacks can curb your appetite and prevent overeating during main meals. Discover the magic of nutrient-dense snacks, where foods like nuts, seeds, and yogurt provide a concentrated source of vitamins and minerals.

Explore creative snack ideas that cater to various dietary preferences, from crunchy veggie sticks and hummus to satisfying energy balls made with natural ingredients. Learn the importance of mindful snacking, allowing yourself to savor the flavors and sensations of each bite, ultimately promoting better digestion and satisfaction.

Section 3: The Mindful Plate: A Wholesome Approach to Balanced Eating

Prepare to transform your relationship with food through the art of mindful eating. In this section, we delve into the practice of mindfulness as it relates to your dietary choices, exploring how cultivating awareness can lead to a more fulfilling and balanced approach to nourishment.

Embark on a journey of conscious eating, where each meal becomes an opportunity to savor the flavors, textures, and aromas of your food. Learn how to differentiate between physical and emotional hunger, allowing you to make choices that truly satisfy your body's needs.

Explore the practice of mindful portion control, understanding how tuning in to your body's cues can prevent overeating and promote optimal digestion. Discover the joy of eating without distractions, giving yourself the gift of presence and connection with your food.

As you navigate this chapter, remember that building healthy habits is a journey of self-care and empowerment. Embrace the power of meal planning, the art of smart snacking, and the transformative practice of mindful eating. Let these strategies become the cornerstone of your wellness journey, guiding you toward a lifetime of balanced nourishment and vitality.

Chapter 6: Special Dietary Considerations: Navigating the Diverse Landscape of Nutritional Needs

Welcome to a chapter that celebrates the unique tapestry of dietary choices, from vegetarian and vegan lifestyles to managing food allergies and intolerances. "Special Dietary Considerations" invites you to explore the world of diverse nutritional needs, offering insights and strategies to embrace a nourishing and inclusive approach to food.

Section 1: Embracing Plant-Based Diets: Nurturing Nutritional Well-Being

Imagine a world where plants take center stage on your plate, shaping your health and values. In this section, we delve into the vibrant realm of plant-based diets, from vegetarian to vegan lifestyles, uncovering the rich tapestry of benefits and challenges they offer.

Embark on a journey of nutritional exploration as we delve into the world of vegetarianism. Learn how to source essential nutrients like protein, iron, and B vitamins from plant-based foods, all while crafting meals that celebrate the beauty of nature's bounty.

Venture further into the realm of veganism, where a commitment to avoiding all animal products shapes both your dietary choices and your ethical compass. Explore the art of creating balanced and diverse meals that provide the nutrients your body needs for optimal health.

Section 2: Navigating Food Allergies and Intolerances: Crafting Inclusive Plates

Prepare to explore the intricacies of food allergies and intolerances, as we navigate the world of dietary restrictions with empathy and knowledge. In this section, we uncover the science behind common allergens and intolerances, empowering you to make informed choices while catering to your unique needs.

Delve into the world of gluten sensitivity and celiac disease, understanding the nuances of avoiding gluten while maintaining a balanced diet. Explore the challenges of dairy intolerance and the multitude of dairy alternatives that allow you to enjoy your favorite foods without discomfort.

Uncover strategies for managing nut allergies and sensitivities, as we explore the creative use of seeds and other nutrient-rich alternatives. Learn the art of reading labels and identifying hidden allergens, ensuring that your meals remain safe and satisfying.

Section 3: Inclusivity and Celebration: Cultivating a Welcoming Table

Prepare to celebrate the diversity of dietary choices, as we embrace the power of inclusivity and understanding. In this section, we explore the importance of creating meals that cater to a variety of needs, allowing everyone to partake in the joy of shared nourishment.

Dive into the world of allergen-free cooking, as we learn how to create dishes that are free from common triggers without compromising on flavor and enjoyment. Explore the art of hosting gatherings that cater to diverse dietary needs, ensuring that every guest feels welcome and cherished.

As you navigate this chapter, remember that special dietary considerations are a testament to the rich tapestry of human preferences and needs. Whether you're embracing a plant-based lifestyle, managing allergies, or accommodating sensitivities, your nutritional journey is a celebration of choice, empowerment, and unity.

Chapter 7: The Mind-Body Connection: Exploring the Interplay of Nutrition and Mental Well-Being

Welcome to a chapter that delves into the profound connection between what we eat and how we feel. "The Mind-Body Connection" invites you to explore the intricate relationship between nutrition and mental well-being, uncovering the ways in which our dietary choices influence our mood, cognition, and emotional health.

Section 1: Nourishing the Brain: The Role of Nutrition in Cognitive Function

Imagine food as fuel for your brain, shaping your cognitive abilities and mental clarity. In this section, we embark on a journey through the science of brain nutrition, discovering how specific nutrients influence memory, focus, and overall cognitive function.

Dive into the world of brain-boosting nutrients, from omega-3 fatty acids that support neural connections to antioxidants that protect against oxidative stress. Explore the power of B vitamins in promoting mental agility and learn how hydration plays a vital role in maintaining optimal brain function.

Uncover the role of gut health in brain health, as we explore the gut-brain axis and its influence on mood and cognitive function. Delve into the impact of prebiotics and probiotics on mental well-being, understanding how a balanced gut microbiome can positively affect your mood.

Section 2: Nutrition and Emotional Well-Being: Crafting a Positive Relationship

Prepare to explore the ways in which nutrition influences our emotional well-being, shaping our moods, stress levels, and overall mental resilience. In this section, we delve into the science behind the "food-mood" connection, uncovering how specific nutrients can impact our emotional states.

Embark on a journey into the world of neurotransmitters, those chemical messengers that regulate our emotions and mood. Learn how amino acids like tryptophan and tyrosine play a role in the production of serotonin and dopamine, neurotransmitters that contribute to happiness and motivation.

Discover the power of antioxidants in combating oxidative stress and inflammation, factors that are linked to mood disorders and mental health challenges. Explore the impact of vitamin D on seasonal affective disorder and its role in promoting a positive mood.

Section 3: Mindful Eating and Mental Health: Cultivating a Harmonious Approach

Prepare to transform your relationship with food into a mindful practice that nurtures both body and mind. In this section, we explore the concept of mindful eating and its influence on mental well-being, as well as the role of nutrition in managing conditions like anxiety and depression.

Delve into the practice of eating with awareness, learning how to savor each bite and cultivate a deeper connection with your food. Explore how mindfulness can combat emotional eating and promote healthier relationships with food.

Uncover the impact of nutrients like magnesium, zinc, and omega-3 fatty acids on managing anxiety and depression. Learn about the gut-brain connection and its role in conditions like irritable bowel syndrome (IBS) and how dietary changes can alleviate symptoms.

As you navigate this chapter, remember that the mind-body connection is a journey of empowerment and self-care. By understanding the intricate ways in which nutrition influences our mental well-being, we can make choices that promote cognitive clarity, emotional balance, and overall mental resilience.

Chapter 8: Sustainable Nutrition: Nurturing Your Body and the Planet

Prepare to embark on a journey that transcends personal well-being and extends to the health of our planet. "Sustainable Nutrition" invites you to explore the intricate interplay between our dietary choices and the environment, uncovering the ways in which our food decisions impact not only our bodies but also the world around us.

Section 1: The Environmental Footprint of Diets: From Farm to Table

Imagine every meal as a conversation with the Earth, as we delve into the environmental footprint of different dietary choices. In this section, we explore how our diets contribute to resource consumption, greenhouse gas emissions, and the overall health of our ecosystems.

Dive into the world of carbon footprints, understanding how various diets—ranging from plant-based to animal-centric—impact our planet's health. Explore the role of food production in deforestation, water usage, and biodiversity loss, and learn how sustainable choices can mitigate these effects.

Venture into the realm of food miles, uncovering the hidden costs of transporting food across long distances. Learn the benefits of supporting local and seasonal produce, reducing your carbon footprint and embracing the flavors of your region.

Section 2: Reducing Food Waste: A Pathway to Sustainability

Prepare to explore the issue of food waste, as we uncover the ways in which our consumption patterns contribute to global food loss. In this section, we delve into the art of reducing food waste, not only for the sake of our wallets but also for the health of the planet.

Embark on a journey through the stages of food production, distribution, and consumption, understanding where food waste occurs and how to address it. Learn strategies for mindful meal planning, storage, and repurposing leftovers, all of which contribute to a more sustainable kitchen.

Delve into the role of imperfect produce, exploring how embracing "ugly" fruits and vegetables can reduce waste and support local farmers. Discover the concept of upcycled foods, where ingredients that would otherwise go to waste are transformed into nutritious products, reducing the burden on landfills.

Section 3: The Joy of Mindful Consumption: Nurturing a Green Plate

Prepare to transform your eating habits into a mindful act of planetary stewardship. In this section, we explore how embracing sustainable nutrition is not only an ethical choice but also a deeply satisfying way to engage with your food.

Discover the concept of eco-friendly eating, as we explore plant-based diets and their positive impact on reducing resource consumption and greenhouse gas emissions. Learn about the concept of "flexitarianism," which encourages balanced consumption of both plant and animal-based foods.

Venture into the world of sustainable seafood, as we uncover the importance of choosing seafood options that are not only delicious but also harvested in ways that support ocean health and marine ecosystems. Learn about certification programs that guide consumers toward sustainable choices.

As you navigate this chapter, remember that sustainable nutrition is a powerful act of interconnectedness. By making choices that nourish both your body and the planet, you contribute to a more harmonious and balanced world—one that ensures well-being for generations to come.

Chapter 9: Navigating Challenges and Staying Consistent: Overcoming Obstacles on Your Wellness Journey

Welcome to a chapter that acknowledges the twists and turns that accompany any transformative journey. "Navigating Challenges and Staying Consistent" invites you to explore the common hurdles that can arise on your path to optimal health and provides strategies to overcome them, ensuring your commitment to wellness remains unwavering.

Section 1: The Ebb and Flow of Motivation: Sustaining Your Wellness Drive

Imagine motivation as a flame that needs nurturing to stay alive, as we delve into the nuances of maintaining enthusiasm for your wellness journey. In this section, we explore the cycles of motivation and provide strategies to reignite your passion when the flame wavers.

Embark on a journey of self-awareness, understanding the factors that trigger motivation and the potential pitfalls that can lead to setbacks. Learn how to set achievable goals that keep you engaged and inspired, while also embracing flexibility to adapt to changing circumstances.

Discover the role of support systems, from friends and family to online communities, in providing encouragement and accountability. Explore the art of positive self-talk and mindfulness, as we delve into the power of affirmations and visualization in maintaining a positive mindset.

Section 2: Overcoming Plateaus: Breaking Through Stagnation on Your Journey

Prepare to tackle the challenge of plateaus, those moments when progress seems to stall. In this section, we delve into the reasons behind plateaus and offer strategies to break through these moments of stagnation.

Explore the science behind plateaus, from metabolic adaptations to changes in exercise routines, and learn how to adjust your approach to reignite progress. Discover the benefits of variety, as we delve into the importance of mixing up your workouts and trying new foods to keep your body engaged.

Venture into the world of mindful indulgence, as we explore how occasional treats can actually support your long-term success by preventing feelings of deprivation. Learn how to differentiate between true plateaus and temporary fluctuations, empowering you to stay the course.

Section 3: Navigating Social and Lifestyle Challenges: Balancing Wellness and Enjoyment

Prepare to navigate the social and lifestyle challenges that can arise when your wellness journey intersects with your daily life. In this section, we explore strategies to navigate social gatherings, travel, and other lifestyle factors without compromising your commitment to well-being.

Embark on a journey of effective communication, as we learn how to express your dietary preferences and needs to friends, family, and hosts. Discover strategies for making healthy choices while dining out or traveling, from researching restaurant menus to packing nutrient-dense snacks.

Delve into the art of mindful moderation, understanding that enjoying special occasions and indulging in treats can coexist with your commitment to wellness. Learn to strike a balance between maintaining your routine and embracing the spontaneity and joy that life offers.

As you navigate this chapter, remember that challenges are a natural part of any journey, and the way you navigate them can shape your ultimate success. By acknowledging the hurdles and implementing strategies to overcome them, you're poised to stay consistent and resilient on your path to optimal health.

Chapter 10: Your Wellness Roadmap: Crafting a Lifetime of Health and Fulfillment

Welcome to the culminating chapter of your journey, where we synthesize the wisdom gained throughout this book into a comprehensive wellness roadmap. "Your Wellness Roadmap" invites you to reflect on your achievements, set intentions for the future, and embrace a holistic approach to health that extends beyond the pages of this guide.

Section 1: Reflecting on Your Progress: Celebrating Achievements

Imagine this chapter as a mirror that reflects your growth, resilience, and dedication to your well-being. In this section, we guide you through a reflection on your journey, encouraging you to celebrate your achievements and the positive changes you've experienced.

Embark on a journey of gratitude, acknowledging the steps you've taken and the milestones you've reached. Celebrate not only the visible changes but also the newfound energy, mental clarity, and overall sense of well-being that you've cultivated.

Dive into the art of self-compassion, recognizing that setbacks and challenges are part of any journey. Learn how to embrace these moments with kindness, understanding that they are opportunities for growth and learning.

Section 2: Setting Intentions: Mapping Your Future Wellness

Prepare to set your compass toward a future of continued growth and well-being. In this section, we explore the power of setting intentions and goals that align with your values, ensuring that your wellness journey remains vibrant and purposeful.

Embark on a journey of envisioning, imagining the kind of life you want to lead and the health and vitality that support your aspirations. Learn to set SMART goals—Specific, Measurable, Achievable, Relevant, and Time-bound—that provide a clear roadmap for your actions.

Venture into the world of holistic well-being, understanding that your health extends beyond just physical vitality. Explore intentions related to mental health, emotional balance, relationships, and personal fulfillment, embracing a multidimensional approach to your wellness journey.

Section 3: Embracing Lifelong Learning: Nourishing Your Mind and Body

Prepare to cultivate a mindset of curiosity and lifelong learning, as we explore the importance of continuing to nourish both your mind and body. In this section, we delve into the art of staying informed, open-minded, and adaptive in your approach to well-being.

Embark on a journey of exploration, as we encourage you to seek out new information, trends, and research that align with your wellness goals. Learn to critically evaluate sources and embrace evidence-based practices that support your journey.

Delve into the art of experimentation, as we encourage you to continue trying new foods, workouts, and wellness practices to keep your routine fresh and engaging. Explore the concept of bioindividuality, understanding that what works for one person may not work for another, and embrace the journey of self-discovery.

As you navigate this chapter, remember that your wellness journey is a lifelong adventure that evolves with you. By reflecting on your progress, setting intentions, and embracing ongoing learning, you're poised to craft a future of health, fulfillment, and purpose that extends far beyond the confines of these pages.

Chapter 11: Sharing Your Wellness Journey: Inspiring Others and Creating Impact

Welcome to a chapter that celebrates the power of connection and influence that comes from sharing your wellness journey. "Sharing Your Wellness Journey" invites you to explore how your personal transformation can inspire others, foster a sense of community, and create a ripple effect of positive change.

Section 1: The Ripple Effect of Sharing: Inspiring Transformation

Imagine your wellness journey as a pebble dropped into a pond, creating ripples that extend far beyond your own experience. In this section, we explore the potential impact of sharing your journey with others, inspiring them to embrace positive changes in their lives.

Embark on a journey of storytelling, as we delve into the art of authentically sharing your challenges, triumphs, and lessons learned. Learn how vulnerability can create connections and relatability, inspiring others to take their own steps toward wellness.

Venture into the world of social influence, as we explore the concept of leading by example. Discover how your commitment to well-being can motivate friends, family, and even acquaintances to make positive changes in their own lives.

Section 2: Building a Supportive Community: Nurturing Connection

Prepare to explore the power of community in your wellness journey, as we uncover the ways in which shared experiences create a sense of belonging and support. In this section, we delve into the importance of finding or creating a community that aligns with your wellness goals.

Dive into the world of online and offline communities, from social media groups to local meetups, that offer a platform for sharing experiences, tips, and encouragement. Learn how these communities can provide a sense of accountability and camaraderie that enhances your journey.

Explore the concept of wellness partnerships, as we encourage you to find a friend, family member, or partner who shares your goals and can journey alongside you. Discover the benefits of mutual motivation, shared challenges, and the joy of celebrating each other's successes.

Section 3: Paying It Forward: Creating Lasting Impact

Prepare to explore how your wellness journey can extend beyond your immediate circle and create a lasting impact in your community and beyond. In this section, we delve into the ways in which you can pay your positive transformation forward.

Embark on a journey of service, as we explore opportunities to volunteer, mentor, or educate others about the benefits of wellness. Discover the fulfillment that comes from supporting others on their journey and contributing to a healthier and happier world.

Delve into the concept of advocacy, as we encourage you to use your voice to raise awareness about wellness-related causes and issues. Explore the power of social media, public speaking, and community involvement in creating positive change on a larger scale.

As you navigate this chapter, remember that your wellness journey is not just personal; it's a story that can inspire, a community that can support, and a movement that can create lasting change. By sharing your transformation and embracing the power of community, you're poised to amplify your impact and leave a positive mark on the world.

Chapter 12: The Ever-Evolving Journey: Embracing Change and Continual Growth

Welcome to a chapter that celebrates the dynamic nature of your wellness journey. "The Ever-Evolving Journey" invites you to explore the concept of growth, adaptability, and lifelong learning as you navigate the twists and turns that life brings your way.

Section 1: Embracing Change as a Constant: Navigating Life's Seasons

Imagine your wellness journey as a river that flows through various landscapes and seasons. In this section, we delve into the concept of change as a constant companion, and we explore how to adapt your wellness practices to different phases of life.

Embark on a journey of self-compassion, as we navigate the challenges that arise when life throws curveballs. Learn how to embrace flexibility in your routines, understanding that maintaining well-being is about balance and adaptability, rather than rigid adherence.

Venture into the world of life transitions, from starting a new job to becoming a parent or navigating retirement. Explore strategies to prioritize your wellness during times of change, finding creative ways to incorporate healthy habits into your evolving daily life.

Section 2: The Art of Lifelong Learning: Cultivating Curiosity

Prepare to explore the importance of embracing a growth mindset in your wellness journey. In this section, we delve into the concept of lifelong learning, as well as the ways in which curiosity can fuel your passion for well-being.

Dive into the world of exploration, as we encourage you to continuously seek out new experiences, foods, activities, and knowledge that enrich your well-being. Learn how adopting a curious attitude can keep your journey fresh, engaging, and invigorating.

Discover the power of setting new challenges and goals, as we explore how the pursuit of mastery can inspire and elevate your wellness journey. Embrace the journey of becoming a perpetual student of your own body, mind, and health, and find joy in each new discovery.

Section 3: Reflection and Integration: A Holistic Approach to Growth

Prepare to reflect on your journey with a lens of integration, embracing the full spectrum of experiences and insights that have shaped your path. In this section, we delve into the art of reflecting on your growth and weaving the lessons into your daily life.

Embark on a journey of self-reflection, as we guide you through practices that encourage introspection and mindfulness. Learn to celebrate not only the successes but also the challenges and setbacks that have contributed to your growth.

Delve into the concept of holistic integration, understanding how the lessons you've learned can influence various areas of your life. Explore how your wellness journey can inform your relationships, career choices, and overall sense of purpose.

As you navigate this chapter, remember that your wellness journey is a lifelong adventure marked by growth, discovery, and transformation. By embracing change, cultivating curiosity, and reflecting on your experiences, you're poised to create a meaningful and vibrant life that continuously evolves in alignment with your values.

Chapter 13: Your Wellness Legacy: Cultivating Lasting Impact and Leaving a Mark

Welcome to a chapter that delves into the legacy you'll leave behind as a result of your wellness journey. "Your Wellness Legacy" invites you to explore how the positive changes you've made can create a lasting impact on your own life, your loved ones, and the world around you.

Section 1: The Ripple Effect of Well-Being: Nurturing Future Generations

Imagine your wellness journey as a torch that illuminates the path for generations to come. In this section, we explore how the choices you make today can shape the well-being of your family, friends, and even future generations.

Embark on a journey of family well-being, understanding how your habits and values can inspire your loved ones to embrace healthier lifestyles. Learn how to create an environment that encourages positive choices, from preparing nourishing meals together to engaging in physical activities as a family.

Venture into the world of education and mentorship, as we explore the ways in which you can inspire and guide others on their own wellness journeys. Discover the joy of passing on your knowledge, experiences, and insights to those who seek guidance and inspiration.

Section 2: Cultivating Social Impact: Wellness as a Catalyst for Change

Prepare to explore how your wellness journey can extend its impact beyond your immediate circle and contribute to positive change in your community and society at large. In this section, we delve into the potential of wellness as a catalyst for social transformation.

Dive into the concept of wellness advocacy, as we explore the ways in which you can use your voice and influence to raise awareness about health-related issues. Learn how to engage in conversations that promote positive change and challenge harmful norms.

Delve into the world of community engagement, from volunteering in health-related initiatives to organizing events that promote wellness education and awareness. Explore the joy of being a driving force behind positive change and a healthier, happier community.

Section 3: Legacy of Mindful Living: A Gift to Future Generations

Prepare to explore the concept of leaving a legacy of mindful living, where your choices become a gift to future generations. In this section, we delve into the ways in which you can create a lasting impact that extends far beyond your own lifetime.

Embark on a journey of environmental stewardship, understanding how sustainable choices and responsible consumption can contribute to a healthier planet for future generations. Learn how reducing your ecological footprint can become part of your wellness legacy.

Discover the power of education and advocacy, as we explore how you can contribute to wellness-focused initiatives, policies, and organizations that will continue to shape the landscape of health and well-being long after you're gone.

As you navigate this chapter, remember that your wellness journey is not just a personal endeavor; it's an opportunity to create a meaningful legacy that ripples through time and space. By nurturing well-being in your family, inspiring change in your community, and advocating for a healthier world, you're poised to leave a positive mark that will be felt for generations to come.

Conclusion: Embracing a Lifelong Journey of Wellness and Fulfillment

As we draw the curtains on this comprehensive journey, it's a moment to reflect on the remarkable path you've traversed—from the inception of your wellness aspirations to the creation of a lasting legacy. "Embracing a Lifelong Journey of Wellness and Fulfillment" encapsulates the essence of your transformation and offers a final perspective to guide you forward.

Reflecting on Your Transformation: A Journey Well-Traveled

Take a moment to look back at the chapters you've explored, the insights you've gained, and the steps you've taken. Your journey has been one of self-discovery, growth, and empowerment. You've not only learned about nutrition and health but also the power of intention, community, and positive change.

Embracing Wellness as a Lifestyle, Not a Destination

Wellness is not a destination you reach and then stop—it's a lifelong journey. Embrace the understanding that your path to well-being is a continuous cycle of growth, self-care, and adaptation. Just as seasons change, so too will your priorities, goals, and challenges. The key is to remain flexible, resilient, and open to learning.

Your Wellness Legacy: Inspiring and Creating Impact

As you move forward, consider the legacy you wish to leave behind. Your choices have a far-reaching impact, from inspiring your loved ones to fostering change in your community and beyond. Your commitment to well-being has the power to shape a healthier, happier world for generations to come.

Continuing Your Path of Growth and Transformation

Remember that you are the author of your wellness journey, and you hold the pen to write the chapters that lie ahead. Embrace curiosity, seek new challenges, and continue to cultivate a mindset of lifelong learning. Your journey will be filled with highs and lows, but each experience will contribute to your growth.

A Message of Gratitude and Encouragement

As we conclude this guide, know that your commitment to well-being is a gift—to yourself, your loved ones, and the world. Embrace your unique journey, cherish your progress, and face the future with the knowledge that you possess the tools to lead a life of vitality, purpose, and fulfillment.

Feel free to revisit any chapter at any time, and remember that your wellness journey is ongoing. As you continue to navigate life's twists and turns, know that you have the wisdom, strength, and resilience to create a life that reflects your values and honors your well-being.

May your journey be marked by a tapestry of joy, growth, and well-being. Embrace each moment as an opportunity for transformation, and let the chapters of your life unfold with purpose and intention.